LOSE WEIGHT DIET FOR LIFE

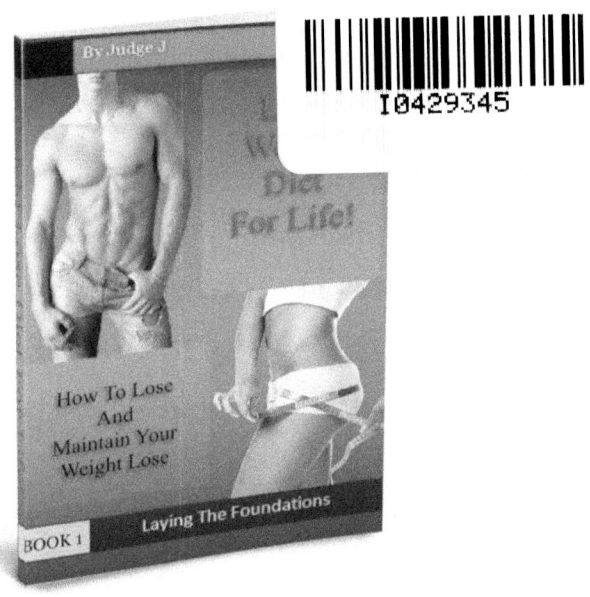

I0429345

'HOW' to LOSE AND MAINTAIN YOUR WEIGHT

By: JUDGE J

Contents:

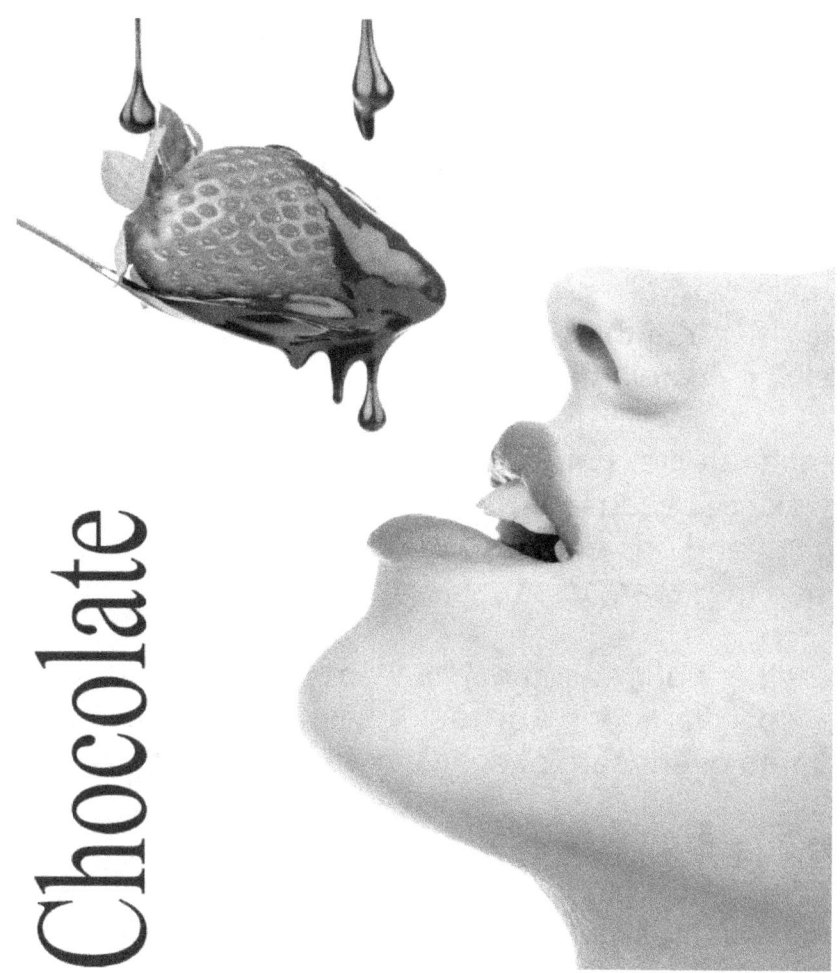

Chocolate

INTRDUCTION

Managing your weight is not the same as *'Going on a diet'*? A diet deals with losing weight and that's it, you are then left to your own devices.

Managing your weight is a strategy in losing and then controlling your weight at a level you wish to maintain...it's all about leading a healthier *'lifestyle'*, not just for you, but for those that share your life too!

There's no greater reason to diet than for your personal health, your welfare, and for those you love around you.

Those who are overweight understand only too well the risks and the possible price that might result from being overweight.

In that sense, being overweight can be compared to smoking, because the risks don't always appear quite so cut and dry, until they reach their own turning point when they want to stop.

Whether your eating habits were born of an addiction to specific foods, or out of emotional needs, or formed over years of conditioned behaviour.

The fact is things won't change much until you understand that you need to alter your eating habits, and your lifestyle choices, before any success can be achieved.

Dieting for most, is nothing more than an endless rapid flip-flopping, or yo-yoing, from one diet to another, with little success.

There is also this ever growing inward desperation that creeps over their confidence, because of their sheer lack of results.

The truth is there are no easy ways to lose weight, and until you decide to forgive yourself, learn from your failures, and get yourself back on the bike after falling off, so to speak... no diet or weight loss plan is going to be successful.

No diet plan is going to make you lose fat by magic; they can't make the pounds disappear, because most don't have a plan.

You will be surprised to learn just how many diets leave out the number 1, most important ingredient, and is setting you up for failure.

Constantly depriving yourself of those things you enjoy eating most, will only lead to more frustration and stress, misery, eventually leading on to negative ways.

Forcing you to comfort eat and the cycle continues.

In order to be able to defeat your weight problem, and the most important, is to learn how your body works, and 'What' you have to do to combat problems you are going to face in the not too distant future.

Putting this step into action right now, will eventually help you to overcome the hurdles you will meet along your journey.

Now I just want to mention the use of scales. People use scales to judge weight lost, this in my opinion is a grave mistake, and one you should be aware of.

There's no doubt that using scales to measure you weight can be your best friend, but in most causes it turns into your own worst enemy, depending on your personal nature?

If you weigh yourself daily in the hope of seeing the scale tick off yet another pound, you're probably dooming yourself to failure before you have started.

You need to understand, and burn this into your memory, when you first start to lose weight your body will try to compensate for the drop in body weight, your body will always try to keep the status-quo.

So your body will increase your body weight one day and let it go on another.

So if you happen to be weighing yourself on a day when your body has increased in weight... then you are going to become very unhappy, depressed, and disappointed.

Try weighing yourself once a week... or use a mirror instead. Also, bear in mind you will lose a lot of water to begin with, not fat, so weighing will more than lightly represent water lose and not body fat.

Try not to get hung-up by weighing yourself to often, leave the scales to once a week.

Dieting flat-out doesn't work, however, a lot of lifestyle changes, if practiced consistently, and aggressively... **_will work_**.

Commonly when people consider starting any form of managing their own weight, things usually end-up going completely wrong for them.

In fact, the truth is that most will be worse off, even putting on more weight when cycling off their diet.

If you really want to gain control over your weight, then there are some very important measures you must adhere to in order to achieve any real success.

This book is the first of many books I have written on the subject of weight loss.

The main reason I wrote it was to help you get you off on the right track, planning your journey so you can't fail.

Weight lose is a voyage through the unknown, I will guild you by the hand through this minefield of confusion, clearing the way ahead onwards to your ultimate goal, burning off your body fat for good.

It's your personal guide, helping to prime you for a new way of life, where the endless daily struggles to control your weight is finally laid down to rest.

There are several things one should prepare oneself for before attempting any form of weight management.

However, before we start this process, we first need to assess and confirm that controlling your weight is something you really want to do.

Do I doubt your sincerity to lose weight... No.
But neither do I want you to have any doubts about your conviction too.

One of the main intentions of writing this book is to get you, the reader, to ask yourself some fundamental questions as to whether or not, you really want to lose and eventually gain some control over your weight to help better your lifestyle.

Also, to bring to your attention the real reasons why you may have already failed to control your weight in the past, and the best ways to help combat and rectify those problems.

But first, below are some very important questions you should be asking ask yourself:

Do you want to lose weight?

Are you ready to lose weight?

Are you prepared to work hard?

Is this really what you want?

These are very important questions that must be answered before embarking on your new healthier lifestyle.

Be as honest as possible, because failure is not an option.

There is something you should understand about people; they are very different to one another. Some people really are strong minded and when they say they want to do something, they do.

But there are the others who are in love with the idea of losing weight, but really **_DON'T_** want to lose weight.

We need to know right now which one of these two different types of people you are.

If you answered **No**, then please come back when you are ready. This may sound harsh, but we both know that this isn't going to work.

However, if you answered **'Yes'** to any of the above questions, then the chances are you are someone who possesses the right personality to get to grips with the fundamentals of mastering their own weight destiny, and a very positive outcome.

And my congratulations for taking your first, tentative steps, plunging yourself towards creating a solid grounding to achieving your goals, and for reading my book!

Now just before we get started on the essential preparation for managing and controlling your weight, we will focus on some preparatory steps first.

You will need to consider these before initiating this very exciting and important journey.
After all, managing your weight truly is a journey - a journey of the body, spirit and mind. And like any journey, you need to prepare before your voyage.

Before taking your first steps into a brand new world and lifestyle. Here are some helpful guidelines, which will preparation you on your epic journey to a better and healthier you.

1 - Drinking lots of water

Drinking lots of water is a component that people looking to manage their weight should do, 'why', because it helps to detoxify and flush out impurities from the body.

If you are already used to drinking lots of water, when it comes time to controlling your weight, then this will have become second nature, which is what you need.

2 - Arranging time to exercise

An important part of the discipline essential for managing your weight involves arranging some time to yourself for some sort of exercise.

It's very important to plan exercise around your daily life. It doesn't mean going down the gym if you don't want too.

Instead do some walking, running, swimming, or cycling for example.

Doing this way ahead of starting your diet, will defiantly help your slide into a better, and more, appropriate mindset.

It's a good habit to get into, making your preparations and ongoing plans a lot easier to cope with.

Some form of exercise is important, because any diet puts stress on your body, which is extremely counterproductive, probably increasing your weight and encouraging you to give-up.

But when you exercise the brain releases endorphins giving you a feeling of joy and happiness, forging you forward to stay the course.

3 - Being persistent

This as to be one of the most important habits you need to form... be 'Persistent' with yourself.

When you first start any enterprise you start off with all the enthusiasm in the world, but this tends to be short lived.

Woven in-between this enthusiasm will be periods when you just can't be bothered to carry on.

If you can battle your way through these phases, these periods of depression become less frequent, if you can't you will give-in and stop.

There's only one way to deal with apathy, be 'Persistent' with yourself stick to your planed routines at all costs.

4 – Exercise

In 2 about, *'arranging time to exercise'* we dealt with time management, how let's take a look at the possibility of exercising, and why you should.

If you hate the idea of doing exercise, then don't worry, because you are not alone.

Most people wouldn't consider this to be their favourite past-time.

However, unfortunately, exercise is an important part of managing your weight. You see when you start on any weight management program; it puts your body under stress.

This can lead to more weight making you feel like quitting.

As I explained above, when you exercise your brain releases endorphins that makes us feel happier, more like training, and you start to lose fat.

The trick with exercise is to start off slowly, with baby steps, stepping-up when you feel you can.

Luckily the following tips will help you to eventually learn to love exercise.

The real trick is to find exercises that you don't mind doing, walking, swimming, cycling, are a few options

you should consider, opposed to hours of sit ups, lunges, or pushing weight in the gym.

Exercise is also important to improve your strength and flexibility.

If you can get to the gym, you will meet like mined people; this will help you to expand your social circle.

As you can see, managing your weight involves a little bit more than just waking up one day and saying, ***"Hey, I need to manage my weight"***.

Perhaps that is the first step; however, in order to actually accomplish some success when it comes to managing your weight, you must prepare yourself first so you are able to take full advantage of your diet.

Managing Your Weight - A Look Back

you are not the first or last person in the world who would love to that control over their weight.

As a matter of fact, there are tens of thousands of people all over the world who would love to get to grips with their out-of-control weight levels.

How you have the opportunity to acquire these techniques and skills to succeed where you once failed.

The harsh truth is that only a select group of people will ever make the move, change their lifestyles, and commit to an all out effort.

You must have questioned yourself many times over in the past... "Do I want to lose weight"? Diets have a negative effect on a subconscious level, usually they are negative and hold that person back.

But you have reached this point in this book that indicates you are prepared to put the time and effort in to reach your goals.

Well-done for being that awesome person that takes action as opposed to wanting to take action.

Looking back in your history, you probably now realize the reasons behind your past failures and gaining control over your weight loss putting it all back on.

Now you at least have some idea of what is required if you are going to get to the end of the line... like building a good solid foundation.

Managing your weight has a mental and physical aspect to it. Yet any activity you put into place ahead of time will produce a better outcome for you.

It's almost as if the influence you exert with your mind will deliver you to the successful outcome you desire.

If you evaluate those who have been successful in managing their own weight, you can't, but help to notice that they all have one thing in common... they were fully aware of what they were getting themselves involved with.

The Advantages of Weight Loss

Let's remember **'Why'** it is you would like to lose some unwanted weight.

It seems like everyone is trying to lose weight today, and there are a number of justified reasons why a person may want to lose their weight.

Of course, there are always going to be horror stories about people who fall into the traps of eating disorders, but for the most part, losing weight is greatly to your advantage.

It's important to start your exercise routines 'BEFORE' you start food reduction, because you will need all your strength and energy to get you started and recover from that effort.

If you haven't fully recovered from your last exercise outing then you want feel like pushing yourself to train, which could turn into a habit.

The most obvious advantage to weight loss is, of course, the health benefits.

When you are heavier than normal, you put our body at risk of developing a number of diseases and conditions, such as diabetes, high blood pressure, high cholesterol, heart disease, and intestinal diseases.

No one wants to suffer from these conditions, but the good news is most of these can be prevented, and more easily treated if you lose weight.

Maintaining a healthy weight is something that you, your family, and your doctor should discuss in order to make the best decisions for your body's health.

There are, however, other advantages to losing weight. First and foremost, when you are of a normal weight, shopping for clothing is more fun and easier, because you actually fit into clothing more readily... it can often be less expensive as well.

When on a weight control program, you learn about healthy eating, which can open up a whole new world of food.

Cooking with healthy, fresh ingredients can be really fun, you can involve others to participate and help you in the kitchen.

You'll be surprised just how your spouse or children will want to get involved, so that the entire family begins to eat more healthy foods.

It also keeps you focused on losing extra weight and maintaining healthy lifestyle.

It also goes without saying; one of the best advantages will be 'How' you begin to feel about yourself after you've lost some weight… Who doesn't want to receive compliments from your family and co-workers?

Who doesn't want to smile at their appearance every day when they look into the mirror?

Of course, for some people, this takes more than losing weight, but it's a good start.

There are a number of other advantages to losing weight too, for example, you will notice how much more energy you have, be better able to play with your children, have a sense of achievement and much, much more.

A balanced diet is a good place to start, but there are also some great stomach exercises to help with this process.

The exercises describe below, will help to gently introduce you to exercising and strengthening your abdominal muscles.

Not only will they strengthen your ads they will also help to reduce belly fat.

If this is your first attempt at exercising then don't worry, because these exercises were designed with you in mind, they are designed to help people slowly work themselves up to more advanced exercises.

Exercise is hard, and won't work overnight, they take time and effort. But if you stick with the program, you will feel the health benefits kicking in.

Once you have mastered these exercises, move on to more advance techniques that will give you more of a challenge.

When doing these exercises, it is important to take it slowly at first, sometimes your enthusiasm can take over, and you may hurt yourself into the barging.

Below are some examples of exercises you can start with. The first two are beginner's level and the third exercise is more advanced.

If you are new to exercises than start off with the first two and move on when you feel they are becoming easier to do.

Vertical Leg Crunch

This is a variation on the traditional crunch that focuses more specifically on reducing belly fat. To begin this exercise, first lie on your back on a flat surface, such as the floor.

Put a mat or towel on the floor to help cushion your spine. Put your hands behind your head, with elbows out far enough that they are out of sight.

Now lift your legs straight up into the air, crossing your ankles and bending your knees slightly. Contract your abdominals and lift your shoulders, head and upper back up to about a thirty degree angle.

Try not to lift with your hands or lead with your head.

You want to do 3x sets of 8x reps per set. If you find that hard to start with simply cut back on the sets and reps.

Long Arm Crunch

For this stomach exercise, remain on the floor with your knees bent and feet flat.

Again put a mat or towel on the floor to help cushion your spine. Lie back and extend your arms straight back on the floor as though you are reaching above your head.

Contract your abs and slowly lift your arms, head, and shoulders, off the floor to about a thirty degree angle, now hold that angle, then slowly lower your shoulders back to the floor.

Repeat for an entire set. Be careful not to lead with your arms, keeping them straight and above your head.

Again you want to do 3x sets of 8x reps per set. If you find that hard to start with simply cut back on the sets and reps.

Reverse Crunch

You will need to stay on your back for this exercise too. As before use a mat or towel to cushion your spine.

Put your arms at your sides with palms facing up to the ceiling. Put your legs in the air so that your knees are bent at ninety degree angles and your hips make about a ninety degree angle with your torso.

Now raise your legs until they are as straight as possible, at the same time, contract your abdominal muscles so that it feels like your belly button is being pulled toward your spine.

Now this is where it gets a little tricky, at the same time you are contracting your abs, gently lift your hips off the floor.

Raise your hips to the height of a few inches, keeping your legs extended straight upward.

Hold this position for a count of 2, then slowly lower your hips back to the floor.

Repeat for an entire set.

Again you want to do 3x sets of 8x reps per set. If you find that hard to start with simply cut back on the sets and reps.

Managing Your Weight - Step by Step

How you understand what kind of person it takes to be successful at managing their own weight, as well as the character traits that individual needs to possess, let's get started with what we need to do to realize success.

What are the most important life changing steps you need to take in order to change your lifestyle?

1. Be Consistent
2. Be Persistent
3. Remain Positive
4. Determination should be your <u>watch</u> word
5. Drink water during the day
6. Start a Food Diary

First and foremost, and without a doubt, the first physical thing you should do is practice being 'Consistent' in all your efforts and in all things.

I know that I keep harping on about this trace, but, believe me when I say...

"I have seen an overwhelming number of people give up when the finishing line is insight".

Remaining consistent and steadfast is so essential to a successful outcome...

'From this day forward try implementing it into your daily schedule'.

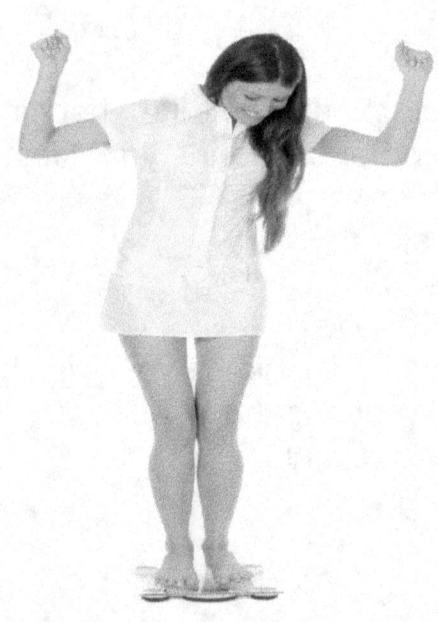

Consistently pushing your boundaries to achieve your goals has many other benefits too.

For one, keeping a constant, flowing effort, towards achieving and accomplishing your goals, will help you build a better, healthier, and, stress free lifestyle, for you and those around you.

Also, the exhilarating feeling of reaching each goal cannot be put into words.

It fills your very soul with energy and delight, something you can't buy, steal or borrow.

It is indescribable, developing self-confidence and admiration from those around you...**well worth the effort**!

Furthermore, eating healthy is essential, and I go into more depth about food in my next book *'The truth About Diets & Weight Loss'*.

There are many benefits to eating healthy apart from managing your weight; it boosts energy levels, which should be at the top of your list.

It's a fact that when fully engaged in controlling your weight, which may involve some dieting, this action will decrease your energy levels.

Decreased energy levels will have a detrimental damaging effect, making it extremely difficult to stay on course.

If your diet is full of carbohydrates, fats, and sugars, then you need to replace them with a well-balanced meal.

Where possible you should always make it a point to eat a balanced mixture of protein and carbohydrates.

Preferably, they should be those with high fibre content, brown rice, oatmeal, whole wheat pasta, and fruits, for example, are all excellent sources.

A word of warning, whatever you do, do not cut out carbohydrates altogether.

Carbohydrates are responsible for fuelling your muscles during exercise, or getting you through a full day's work.

Carbohydrates are also required to help build hormones, so cutting back on carbohydrates will diminish the amount of hormones your body can produce.

This in itself can have a devastating effect on reducing, or burning off excessive fat.

You should endeavour to cut down and replaced carbohydrates with more vegetables.

Cutting out carbohydrates is one of the biggest and dangerous mistakes people tend to make when embarking on any form of food control.

Cutting out carbohydrates will simply push your body into a process of breaking down muscle tissue.

It does this by turning them into amino acids, and then converts them into usable fuel for the brain and the central nervous system.

You are infect, **'<u>Cannibalizing</u>'**, your own body.

Also, the body will convert some of the protein you eat into fuel for the muscles and you don't what this to happen.

Protein is used to repair and build new cells throughout the body.

At this point, you will be losing weight, but it will be water, and muscle tissue, the wrong type of weight to be losing.

There has been some interesting research that shows quite clearly that eating healthy can have a massive effect on reducing your stress levels.

As a matter of fact, it's important to take steps to help relieve stress.

That's because stress can hold you back in so many different ways, making it almost next to impossible to accomplish anything substantial.

It's also well known and documented that stress courses the body to store unused glucose (sugar) in your fat cells.

So even if you change your mind about doing any weight management, you should consider doing some activity to help relieve any stress.

Once you have come to grips with what you need to put into place to sustain a heather lifestyle, you may start to feel like you are now ready to start on a diet plan to manage your weight.

But despite this feeling are you really truly ready, it's best to test if you are truly equipped, or whether your mind is fooling you into thinking you are ready.

It usually takes a couple of weeks of preparation to ensure the right state of mind.

We are all different and develop at different rates, but it is important to make sure you are ready to start your weight management routine.

This will represent a turning point in your life.

Remember, this is not a one-off, managing the ebb and flow of controlling your weight is life changing.

As you begin to get into the preparation process, be sure to dedicate sometime to developing a healthier lifestyle.

It is easy to disregard activities that are particularly directed towards starting a healthy lifestyle, because they usually involve some form of activity.

However, by dedicating time and energy in the early stages of this process, you will find yourself developing a better, more positive outlook.

In addition, starting a healthy lifestyle from the off, will not only help increase your energy levels, but it will have you looking radiant too.

In just a short period of time, simply by sticking to your tasks, eating healthy and starting a healthy lifestyle, you will reach a point when you feel more positive about starting your weight management program.

And you will do it in a quicker time too, and you will be in a better, more positive, state of mind.

You will know when the time is right for you, that's the time to take action.

But for most people it typically takes a couple of weeks of focus and preparation, to reach this stage.

However, time will fly by before you know it.

You should select a date to start your preparations now, calculate a date that falls around two weeks later.

By doing this now, you are giving yourself plenty of time to prepare yourself for what's coming.

This will prepare your body, spirit, and mind, for your journey ahead, total harmony, fully prepared to manage your weight!

Rules to Consider Whilst Preparing to Manage Your Weight

Having said *'yes'* to the questions posed earlier in this book, I can assume that you are a self-reliant and self-determined, person.

Many times these character traits can be brought out of an individual when certain rules are recognized, which command these attributes.

This section will go into particular rules that have been designed purposefully to promote these specific attributes.

Since preparing for the day when you will start your weight control managing routines may take some time and energy to get ready, many of these guidelines can be entrenched in your mind during this preparation period of time.

Since you will possibly be spending around two weeks on preparing, you should have some great opportunities to implement and dedicate sometime to these rules.

Whilst remaining consistent in your tasks, remember to drink lots of water, it's important not to let your body become dehydrated, keeping it refreshed.

If you feel thirsty, then it's too late your body is dehydrated.

I would suggest that you sip water throughout the day, small amounts, but constant.

In addition, you will get better results and feel better about yourself, especially when it comes closer to the time you actually start the process of managing your weight.

Also during this period of preparation, you should keep a journal.

Celebrating milestones when they are reached, you know it is amazing just how these early steps can play such a vital role in the larger picture.

If you believe yourself to be a self-reliant person, you probably won't find it too hard to adopt these rules into your regimented schedule.

In addition, if you actually do keep a journal and celebrate milestones, this will help promote positive feelings of achievement when realizing your goals.

This is a great way of keeping positive and more able to accept your up and coming journey ahead.

In addition, you must bear in mind your commitment to starting a healthier lifestyle.

It is likely that this will need another level of concentration in order to truly start your healthy lifestyle.

During this period of preparation, you will find a little bit of focus will help you go the distance.

Whilst you are working on increasing energy and looking good, you should keep your outlook as positive as possible.

It's important to make sure you retain this mindset, as we all waiver from time to time.

Remaining positive and upbeat will help keep you from becoming discouraged and faltering, before you get the opportunity to begin your weight management routine.

As you can see, it does really take a self-determined person to accomplish the final goal of managing their weight.

Although it is not impossible to reach some level of control over your weight, it's important to keep your guard-up.

I can honestly say it's impossible to maintain any real long term effect, without your determination to remain positive at all times.

Only by preparing your mindset in a positive manner can result in achieving success...

You must remaining faithful and committed to your goals, it's the only way forward to realising your end goals.

With a pledge to fully prepare yourself, you will prevail.

When I asked you the following questions...

Do you want to lose weight?

Are you ready to lose weight?

Are you prepared to work hard?

Is this really what you want?

You replied **'yes'**. Now you understand **'Why'** you answered 'Yes'.

It's because deep inside yourself there was this determined, self-reliant, person trying to get out.

Now is the time to believe in yourself and your ability to finally get yourself into a program to succeed.

You have the very characteristics that will guide you toward your ultimate success and finally gaining that control over your weight you have always wanted.

Just remember to remain consistent in your efforts, eat healthily and get started on that healthy lifestyle...

And you will be a success in no time at all!

The Easiest Way to Manage Your Weight

There are a variety of different ways people can go about managing their weight.

As you will know by now, preparation is Key.

Being prepared is the way forward; it will give you the tools you need to cope with the journey ahead.

Following are some simple instructions that will help guide you through your first two weeks, getting yourself into that working mindset.

First off, you should be drinking lots of water, not because water helps lose weight that is a complete myth... if drinking water helped you to lose body fat there wouldn't be any obesity.

But it does have some additional benefits. It will help flush out toxins from your body.

Drinking water helps to detoxify your body, toxins that build-up in your body will interfere with the process of weight loss.

And flushing out these toxins will also leave you feeling a lot healthier in the process.

Training and dieting will dehydrate you very quickly, so taking in more water now will get you into the habit of drinking more.

So it's important to get rid of and detoxify your body before you begin the process of weight control.

One of the best habits you should learn to follow, right at the beginning of your preparation period, is to drink water BEFORE you eat your meal.

The reason behind this idea is this, drinking water before eating, adds volume to the food you eat.

This will make you feel full quicker and therefore, you eat less.

You should have also start to arrange sometime for your exercise routines, as this will help you organize your day-to-day activities.

The first two weeks should be designated to your need to learn **'how'** to fit all this new activity around your daily routine.

Remember to focus on remaining consistent in your actions, eating healthy, starting a healthier lifestyle.

Keep your mind focused on what we are trying to achieve here.

The emphasis must be on preparing yourself for a change in not just your lifestyle, but those around you to.

This will be ultimately easier than throwing yourself into the deep-end and failing to achieve any of your goals.
You must be sure not to avoid this stage, or it certainly will be hard going for you.

You should always prepare yourself for success and not disappointment.

It's important that you have a head start on this process, feeling better about yourself, improving your lifestyle, as well as boosting your energy.

This grounding will help you seamlessly slip into your new existence, controlling weight and helping you to relieve any stress.

This is all extremely critical to achieving your life long goals.

The great thing about this process, not only will it help you to formulate a better start for your weight management.

But at the end of two weeks, you will have already begun to feel the increase in your energy levels, feeling a lot more positive, and looking great too.

Frequently people incorrectly believe that it is really hard, or even impossible, to gain success in weight management.

But, it really is a lot simpler if you prepare yourself first.

Finding yourself in a new situation that you don't feel comfortable in, or you are struggling to come to terms with, the up-evil, are doomed to failure from the beginning.

If you wholly commit to avoiding cutting corners in the preparation stage and adhere to the work involved, you are basically assured of success.

To summarize, when it comes to controlling your weight, the simplest way is to implement all the steps in this book.

But do avoid rushing through this process, it's not worth it, or you will just end up spending more time than you ultimately needed to.

It really is a simple cause of being properly prepared right from the beginning.

The truth is that 2 weeks does not represent a huge investment of time.

But preparing for an event that will have a major impact on your life is time well spent.

Your dedication and investment in time preparing yourself mentally and physically will have you managing your weight before you even know it!

Managing Your Weight For Free

Sadly, most people think that any form of training is going to involve a lot of expense.

There is a lot of misconception surrounding this subject, but this couldn't be further from the truth.

'Yes' there is some expense involved, but how much really depends upon you.

If you wear the top of the line clothing, shoes, etc, then it's going to cost you, but there's no reason for training to any more expensive than it needs too.

Neither is it necessary to buy any gym equipment, your training can be done on a ... **Shoestring**?

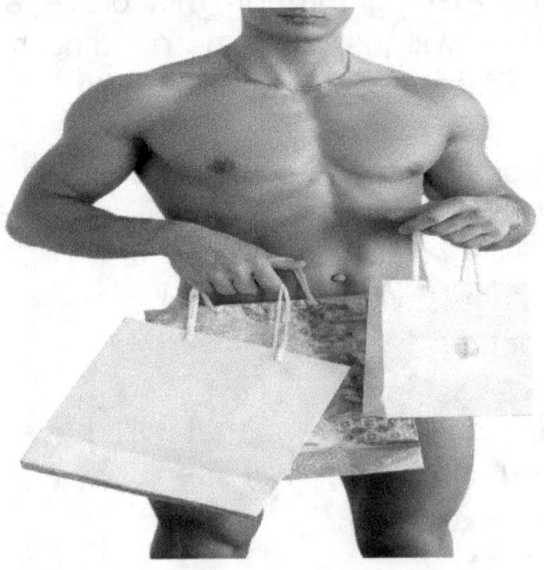

This information generally gets passed around by individuals who are more interested in making an impression with their looks, instead of concentrating on their training.

But when it comes to buying clothing or gym equipment, it is of course your chose.

The problem with this type of information, it can put people off getting started, because they feel it's out of their budget range.

Don't get side tracked by others, start with the bare minimum and acquire them were, and when you need too.

There is no need for you to spend lots of money, because you have everything you need around you...right now!

For example, go for a walk or run around your local park, use your stairs at home to run or walk, up and down, 8 times for about 6 sets.

Buy a second-hand push bike, and go for bike rides, go swimming at your local pool, and **'Why'** you'll at it.

'Why' not involve the family too... getting the idea.

Nice shiny, bells and whistles are not things you should be considering; instead, you should be concentrating on, eating healthy and starting a healthier lifestyle... that's what's really important.

The trick is to find an activity that will allow you to move, slowly at first, and then you can pick-up the pace to what you feel is right for you.

Remember to always remain constant and positive, in your actions and outlook and you will achieve the success you desire.

The greatest piece of advice I or any other fitness instructor can give you, is to keep your centre of attention on your goals, this must always be uppermost in your mind.

Remembering to be consistent, eating healthy, and starting that healthy lifestyle... these are the things you should be concentrating your efforts on.

Take a step back and take a close look at anything you are spending money on, and ask yourself this question... *"Do I really need this "*?

To remain consistent and stick to your tasks is relatively inexpensive and should not cost you a lot of money.

Remember, your main goal is to get better results, and this can be attained without splashing out lots of cash.

And contrary to what you believe eating healthy also does not need to be pricey either... And believe it or not, but it usually takes a lot more money to eat unhealthy.

To help you cut down on the money you may spend on the wrong foods, I'm offering you the opportunity to get my **'FREE'** Healthy Recipes Book, copy this link into your browser...
http://eepurl.com/ct1GMH

The primary reason you should be focusing on eating healthy is to boost your energy levels, which will help you to recover a lot more quickly from the stress of being on a diet, doing exercise, and increasing your immune system.

At this stage, you shouldn't be focusing on expensive equipment, or an expensive gym membership.

Your sole purpose should be on implementing more movement into your daily routine.

And getting yourself ready to embark upon your weight loss, and weight management, program.

Preparing yourself first, getting into the right routines, and keeping a positive frame of mind, will see you reaping the rewards.

Bottom line, you need to focus on your objectives and forget about spending money on unnecessary trivia.

Knowing how your emotions influence your decisions will help enable you to manage and accomplish your objective a lot easer ... making managing your weight a pushover.

Managing Your Weight in Everyday Life

Managing your weight must become natural way of life for you. You can incorporate into your life in a variety of different ways.

Managing or controlling your weight, does require a shift in the way you think.

In order to get to grips with any form of weight control, you must develop a self-reliant nature... this is a quality that is critical to your success.

But luckily for us this can be developed during your initial stages of this program.

The more you exert this quality, the stronger it will become.

Managing your weight is more than just controlling your weight; it really is a way of life, a beneficial addition to your lifestyle.

As can be seen, to accomplish these objectives you must possess a positive attribute, but thankfully, it something you can learn to develop.

Drinking lots of water, arranging time for exercise, and always remaining persistent, can sometimes be seen as acts that go beyond what's needed to gain control over your weight.

What I love about this program, even though we are directing our attention to controlling your weight, it can be used in other areas of your life too.

Do you faintly recall at the opening of this book when you were asked you to answer the following questions:

Do you want to lose weight?

Are you ready to lose weight?

Are you prepared to work hard?

Is this really what you want?

These are lifestyle options, and they are questions calling on the virtues that verify whether, or not, you have enough enthusiasm to be able to manage your weight.

When you answered **'Yes'** to the above questions, you were not just substantiating that you possess the ability to manage your weight, but rather, you were validating you wanted to change your lifestyle.

By recognizing the role that these character traits play in your life decisions, you are acknowledging the role that managing your weight will play in life in the future.

No one says that managing your weight is going to be easy.

On the contrary, if it were easy, then there would be no obesity in the world today, and you wouldn't be reading this book

As we travel through life, we all have to make changes; some are easy, whereas some will be difficult.

Managing your weight is no exception to this rule, from this point onwards; all your actions will take a lot of dedication on your side.

But the rewards can be far more satisfying and far-reaching.

Way beyond anything you could have ever imagined right now.

Congratulations on taking the plunge, your new lifestyle awaits you!

Strategies to Help Manage Your Weight

If you had answered **"No"** to the following question:
Do you want to lose weight?

Then you are probably the type of person who likes the idea of being able to lose and control their weight.

But in reality, they don't want to go through the process of changes that will be required in order to achieve this goal.

If you are that sort of a person, were losing and controlling your weight is really important to you.
But just can't bring yourself around to applying the strategies laid down in this book.

Maybe you need more time to implement the above changes into your lifestyle, and then come back to the possibility at a later date.

Diet writers always assume that all their readers want to lose weight.

But like somebody keeps repeating *"I want to stop smoking"*, but when asked if they truly want to stop smoking, they usually answer...***"Not really"***.

In these cases, smokers always fail to stop smoking.

If you truly want to lose weight and get control over your weight for the rest of your life, you must have a burning desire for this to happen.

Every time you fail to reach your goals, you put yourself into a negative situation that will impact on every attempt you make now and in the future.

Remaining positive, being consistent, and applying your new lifestyle, are all key factors in the process of learning to take control of your weight loss management.

But more importantly your future success.

However, if you answered **'Yes'** to this question, then you need to start preparing yourself for that new lease of life, now, today.

Remember to start by drinking lots of water, water is important as your body is made up mainly of water, and during exercise, you will lose more than normal through sweating.

You need to remember that this water loss will reflect in your weight loss measurements, but when drinking water, a cup of tea, coffee, or any other fluids will put this extra weight loss back on.

Also, water will help to detoxify your body getting rid of harmful toxins from your body.

Next you need to arrange some spare time to dedicate to your new exercise routines.

This is a necessary strategy when preparing an overall plan, which will help in your weight loss program.

Bending, stretching, reaching, walking, cycling, gentle jogging, can all be implemented easily into your daily routine, reaping the benefits of movement.

We are advocating movement here not endurance.

It's important to start slowly and build your way up to a more advanced level.

However, it must be said it's not that important to reach any form of an advanced level...unless you are planning to run a marathon?

Many people get mixed up with what's meant by fitness, and levels of endurance, they are not the same.
It's important to train to bring up your levels of fitness and flexibility.

Fitness is a measurement, which measures how long it that's your heart to return back to normal rhythmic beating, after doing a set amount of energetic exercise.

Endurance, on the other-hand, is the ability to keep going were others would have given-up.

Remember not to run before you can walk, you need to increase your fitness levels first.

Now start thinking about a healthier ways of eating.

Start by cutting down on all the rubbish and unnecessary carbohydrates, like chips, chocolate's, cakes, etc. your eating in your everyday diet.

Yes we know that cutting out all the nice foods you like to eat is going to be hard, but look at it in this way... all that nice food is slowly putting on the weight and killing you.

I'm not saying that you cannot eat any of the above, but just once in awhile, moderation is the key here.

In fact, use these as a nice treat for being good and sticking to a well-balanced meal instead of all that unnecessary carbohydrate.

It's not just a question of cutting back on carbohydrates, but in the process, you will also be cutting back on sugars, fats, and processed foods.

More about the good, bad and ugly foods in my next book... *'The Truth About Weight Lose'*.

Last but not least, also stride to remain **'Positive'** and be **'Persistent'**, in all you do.

These are absolutely vital to ensure you are successful, but the more you practice them the more fixed they become in your daily life.

They may seem like an inconsequential step.

However, without your ability to maintain your focus on accomplishing your objectives, and remaining positive, even when things are not going you way, you may find those well laid out long-term plans, regardless of validity, failing.

Once you have fully implemented all the above traits into your new lifestyle, you will begin to see their benefits.

Not only will these strategies help you to plan a long-term approach to losing and maintaining your weight, but it will also bubble over into your everyday existence.

This will empower a better healthier, and more positive, outlook on your life.

This will of course have some impact upon everyone around you, your loved ones, friends, and those you meet along your life's journey ... well worth all this effort!

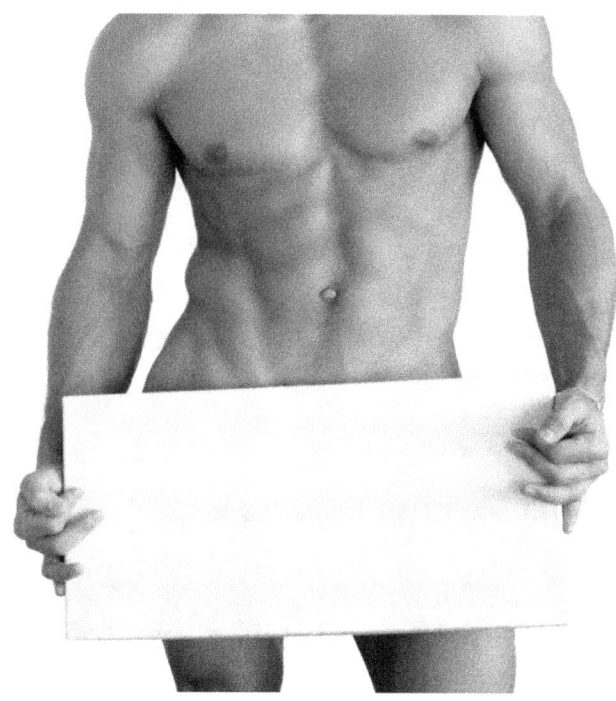

Some Tips to help you on your way

Once you have decided to commit yourself to your

weight management program, there are a number of things you can implement to help reduce your weight, and eventually control your weight better.

The following **Tips** are a few of my suggestions that will help you prepare yourself for your journey ahead:

** Eat your breakfast.

Your body has been asleep for **8hrs** or more, and during these 8hrs; you haven't eaten or drank a thing. Your body needs to replace the protein it's used during the night, to replace, or repair the cells in your body.

You will also be dehydrated too, so replacing these fluids are vitally important to your overall health.

Try combining eggs with melon for breakfast. If you are trying to come up with a breakfast for your diet, then you should try eating melon and eggs.

It's best if you eat the melon first?

But **'Why'** eat Melons with your eggs?

This is because Melons are packed with vitamins, as well as fibre and water, which can give you the feeling of being full, therefore, reducing the amount of food you eat.

And the idea behind eating the eggs after eating the melon is simple...

Eggs are excellent at breaking down the carbohydrates and proteins in the melon, which ads the digestive system to absorb them better.

Tip: I suggest you boil your eggs to reduce the calories.

Tip: If you do slip and find yourself eating a rasher of bacon, for example, eat some 'Avocado', because it has the ability to absorb fat and carry it out of your system.

** If you like aerobic exercise.

You should grab a partner and have a blast with one of the basic aerobic videos... have some fun!

Or, simply go out for a walk and enjoy spending some time together.

If you are finding it difficult to do any walking, then why not consider buying a jogging board?

These padded boards will make running, jumping, or walking in place, less stressful on your knees and joints.

Staying motivated if you hate exercising can be hard, but set goals and don't quit.

You need to exercise as well as diet if you really want to lose weight.

I know you don't want to hear that word 'Exercise', but try making exercise fun and it won't seem like such a chore.

** Start eating healthier.

Reduce the amount of sweets, carbohydrates or junk food you eat.

If you can't go without a snack, try reaching for an apple, an orange, or a fistful of mixed nuts, instead of that chocolate bar or bag of chips.

Reduce calories slowly, don't just reduce by 2000 cal or so a day.

Because you could be putting your body into *'Starvation mode', that's* when your body starts to cannibalize its muscles.

This is a dangerous and unnecessary state to get yourself into, when you can reduce your calories by only 200 cal at the time.

This will help to reduce fat levels, but more importantly, maintain muscle mass.

It's also important to keep as much muscle mass, as possible, as muscle acts like a furnace, burning off calories and reducing fat levels.

Muscles burns more fat than any other process known today.

** keep a journal and celebrate milestones.

This will promote a feeling of achievement when realizing your goals.

It's also important to remember where you have been, and what you did a few months ago.

As you tweak your weight management program, you may inadvertently move in the wrong direction, and then need to revert to what you were doing a few months ago.

Without a Journal you may not remember.

As you adopt these tips in your everyday strategy, you will discover many new benefits along the way.

Following are some you will discover along your journey.

** As you maintain consistency in your strategies.

You will begin getting better results and feeling better within yourself.

** Eating healthy will result in a boost of energy.

It will also increase your feeling of well-being and in your fat burning efforts too.

** As you work towards building a healthy lifestyle.

As time goes by, you will begin to notice a growing positive attitude to life, a better outlook, and you will begin looking and feeling more radiant too.

** You will also notice that your improved lifestyle will help to reduce stress.

This will not only be a huge benefit to yourself, but for those around you too.

Reducing any stress will of course help you remain on course with your diet, but it will help reduce weight too.

Because stress is one of the main courses of weight gain.

These are just some of the advantages that occur when you embark on your journey to get ultimate control over your weight management.

** There is no need for you to spend lots of money managing your weight.

Because you have everything you need around you, right now? You don't need any equipment to lose weight.

** Managing your weight is no more than a state of mind.

Without the right mindset, you will keep on the same path has you are now... is that what you really what?

** Remain constant in everything you do.

Remain as positive and constant, in your outlook has you can, and you will achieve your success.

** Take pictures of yourself.

Prior to starting your diet program, you should take a picture of yourself.

By doing this, you would have a picture that you can compare yourself to after weeks of losing weight.

This can make you more motivated, and ensure that you stay on track.

Once you adopt the tips contained above, you will be well on your way to achieving your desired weight.

Be sure to allow yourself around 2 weeks to prepare yourself for the necessary changes.

The tips above should be your starting point.

One more thing

More about Keeping a Journal or *'Food Diary'*.

Before starting on your weight loss program, one of the smartest, and easiest steps you can make, is to keep a **'Food Diary'**.

A food diary is a notebook in, which you record your daily food and calorie intake.

You can keep track of a number of things in your food diary, or you can keep it simple, but in either case, this is a great way in, which to help yourself stick to your weight loss plan.

There are a number of pieces of information you can record in your food diary. First, consider just listing your daily menu.

This will help you actually see what you eat on any given day, week, or month. From this data, you may notice patterns of unhealthy eating that you have never identified before.

You may also like to record the amount of calories, protein, fibre, fat, and other nutrients you consumed during the day.

You could also record your portion sizes too.

If you truly want to use diary format, you can also list the reasons you're eating, other than hunger, the cravings you are experiencing, and your feelings about your diet on any given day.

It's your diary, so do what is right for you.

When you start a food diary, keep in mind that you don't have to keep a conventional journal by your bedside, under lock and key.

You can use whatever kind of recording or writing tools you like best.

For some people, the traditional journal, or a plain notebook works fine. Also, think about keeping a food diary on your computer.

Simply open up a word processing program and keep the icon on your desktop.

Others like to use Excel, or other data entry programs, which help quite a lot when it comes to adding totals at the end of the day.

You can keep your food diary on a laptop or palm pilot, or slip a notebook into your bag during the day, whatever works best for your lifestyle.

Remember to update your food diary on a daily basis, and review it at the end of each week so you can track your progress.

You should also note in your diary when you hit certain weight loss goals, or when you gain weight, because the causes can be easily seen, and rectified.

You can share your diary with professionals, who can use this information to check-out the state of your health.

Food diaries work great for many people, so you should consider starting one today; as your diary may become your best friend.

After you have gone through all the points in this book, you will have a better understanding of what's involved in getting total control over your weight.

Now you can put together a complete weight management strategy.

You should by now be familiar with every one of the steps required for you to start building your fat burning program.

You have already taken the most vital step toward managing your weight by educating yourself by reading this book.

If you feel that this process may be a little overwhelming, then think about finding a friend with similar goals to yourself.

Many times the *'buddy system'* can work out well when needing an extra boost of confidence, help, or assistance when approaching a goal that requires a helping hand.

Even though you will eventually manage your own weight program, it helps to be able to join another person with similar aspirations to talk about up and coming challenges together.

Just be conscious in your choose of friends, staying clear of those who are indifferent, as they may ultimately undermined or discourage you altogether.

Conclusion

Sadly, there are literally millions of people all over the globe every week that start some form of diet.

Some manage their weight very well, but most fail this task despite all their efforts.

But you have to understand that losing weight is only the beginning of the weight loss story.

The real battle begins when it comes to maintaining the level reached during your weight loss period.

First you need to lose it, and then you need to keep it off?

To begin with losing weight is a physical effort and once all of this physical effort as securely been put into place, it's down to the psychological battle of keeping it off.

I wrote this book in order to bridge this gap between the physical effort and the psychological battle.

But unlike others, I have discovered over the years that most effective way to win this psychological battle is to begin this psychological training first.

This way, not only as the psychological foundation been laid, but during the actual process of losing weight, the process gets reinforced and becomes your way of life, then and only then, will you have finally cracked it...

Judge J

Just before I finish, I would like to stress the point about preparing and remaining as safe as possible during any activity you embark upon.

First off; physical activity is generally safe for everyone. People who are physically fit have **less** chance of injury than those who are not fit.

So start slowly and increase when you feel you are able to do so without injuring yourself.

The health benefits you gain from being active are far greater than the chances of getting hurt... being *inactive* is definitely not good for your health.

Here are some things you can do to stay safe while you are active:

If you haven't been active in a while, start off slowly, ramping up the fitter you get.

Learn about the types and amounts of activity that are right for you.

Choose activities that are appropriate for your fitness level.

Build up the time you spend before switching to activities that take more effort.

Use the right safety gear and sports equipment.

Choose a safe place to do your activity.

See your doctor or health care provider, if you have a health problem.

Don't forget to set your weekly goals, this is an example:

My activity this week - my goal is to do aerobic activities for a total of 2 hours and 30 minutes this week:

What I did	Effort	When I did it and for how long							Total hours or minutes
		Mon	Tue	Wed	Thu	Fri	Sat	Sun	
Walked	Moderate		30 min	30 min		30 min		30 min	2 hours
Biked fast	Vigorous						30 min		30 min
This is the total number of hours or minutes I did these activities this week:									2 hours and 30 min

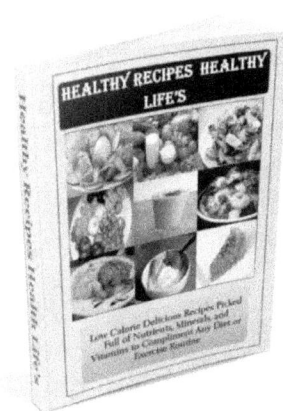

A <u>FREE</u> Health Recipe Book

It Will Make Your Mouth Water
& Keep You Healthy Too

Your 'FREE' gift... **'Healthy Recipes Healthy Life's'** this a free **RECIPE** book packed full of tasty, delicious, filling healthy food recipes, and facts, to help you manage your weight better, after all... 'We Are What We Eat'.

Each recipe contains full calorie count, fat, sodium, cholesterol, fibre, sugar, protein values, for your guidance. And that's not all; find out **'What'** the health benefits of herbals and spices used in these recipes.

Download your **FREE** book; copy this link into your browser: http://eepurl.com/ct1GMH

Further reading...

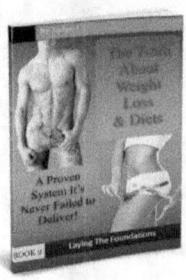

After reading this book, hopefully you should have now started to build that all important foundation. Now you need to build upon that new found knowledge. My **2nd book**...'The Truth About Weight Loss & Diets' addresses and examines the fundamentals of diets.

Going straight onto a diet is asking to fail. It's important to understand the physical and mental restraints a diet will place upon your body and '**How**' to deal with them. **'The Truth About Weight Loss & Diets'** examines these issues and more.

In this very powerful book you will discover '**How**' to succeed where others have failed, expel commonly haled belief and myths, discover which foods are good or bad for you, '**How**' much food you really should be eating, understanding supperments place in dieting, the truth about fat, and so much more.

If you have ever found it hard to lose, or, keep off weight, then don't miss reading this book. To find out more about what this book as to offer, or to grab your own **copy** visit:
http://mybooksupply.com/wp/the-truth-about-weight-lose

*If you enjoyed reading my work, please feel free to check out my other book titles, visit my **Website** at: http://mybooksupply.com*

You can also follow me on –

'Twitter': @hotwealth
'LinkedIn': **http://uk.linkedin.com/in/judgej**
'Facebook': https://www.facebook.com/pages/Lose-weight-manage-weight/343091449182861

'Why' Not Get Your 'Free' Health App – Now

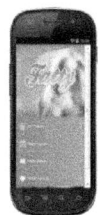 Keep yourself up-to-date with our Free *HealthApp'*... 'YourHealthCoach' Copy the <u>link</u> <u>below</u> to visit the **'Google Play Store'** now - for your 'Free Health App' download...

https://play.google.com/store/apps/details?id=com.squee zemobi.yourhealthcoach

We wish you the best of luck in building your own weight management system!

And I look forward to helping you explore, expand, and develop your weight management strategies in my next book... *My personal wishes in all your endeavours!*

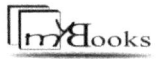